You can do it!

David Madow

IMPRESS THE WORLD WITH YOUR BODY IN SEVEN DAYS

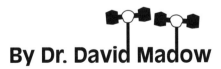

By Dr. David Madow

MADOW BOOKS

Madow, Dr. David

Impress the World With Your Body in Seven Days / David Madow

ISBN 13: 978-0-615-15401-5

Acknowledgements:

Thanks to Dr. Robert Bennett, my physiology professor who introduced me to the world of aerobic exercise. You may not remember me, but you changed my life. My parents, Selvin and Lois Madow, thank you for everything. My children, Lauren and Evan Madow, you two are the greatest. Yoko Okamoto, for all of your support, you know you will always be special to me. Dr. Richard Madow, I couldn't have done all of this without you! Dr. Marshall Madow, follow your dreams my man. Dr. and Mrs. Paul Schenker, two role models I have had for my entire life. Simon and Shirley Madow, you are forever in my heart. Dr. Michael Goldstein, Dr. Larry Goldberg and Dr. Lewis Klotzman, three guys who will always continue to keep me skiing hard, biking long and trekking in cool places. David Levin, the strongest guy I know, thanks for everything you have taught me. I will always be your student. Gary Halbert, for teaching me the fine art of putting words down on paper. Elizabeth Schuman and Dorothy Lasky, for helping me put this book together. Guillermo Fernandez, you are a truly talented artist. Harriet Siebert, you have put up with my craziness from the beginning! Sonny Lee, for letting me always plug my computer in at your sushi bar. William Troxell, for giving me a nod at an important time. Ackley, Phil and Jane. And to all of you who are too numerous to mention. You have impacted my life in a big or a small way. You know who you are.

Congratulations!

You've taken the best step toward a new you. Whether you've bought this book or are reading it in the bookstore, you've made a great start.

What is this book about?

- It's about making you stronger, healthier and more confident.

- It's about making you more attractive to the opposite sex!

- It's about getting you to your ideal weight, and not just for a week or month and then slipping back. I'm going to show you how to stay there forever!

- It's about you! It's about helping you become the person that you have dreamed of — even if you think it's beyond your reach.

- Most of all, it's about how to do all of this with a very simple, "SEVEN DAY" formula. If you follow the "SEVEN DAYS," you will see results.

It's Time to Change!

After following "Impress The World With Your Body in Seven Days," here are some of the many terrific changes that you will notice.

⬡ Your Body

Better balance/posture
Bowel regularity
Decreased blood pressure
Fewer injuries resulting
   from weak muscles
Fewer sick days
Healthier appetite
Improved bone density
Improved digestion
Improved immune system
Improved muscle health

Increased energy
Increased life span
Increased metabolism (you burn
   more calories 24 hrs. a day!)
Increased strength
More lean body mass
Reduction in disease
Stronger bones and decreased
   risk of osteoporosis
Weight loss

⬡ Your Appearance

Healthier gums
Healthier hair
Healthier skin
Less bloating

Less tooth decay
More flexibility
Greater muscle definition

⬡ Your Psyche

Better sleep patterns
Improved mental health (no more stress and depression)
Increased confidence

Inside this Book

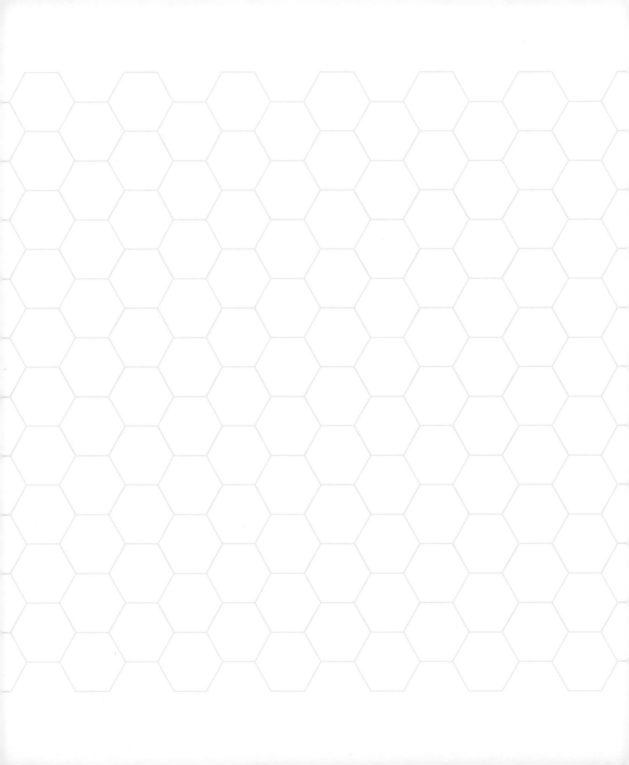

You Probably Knew People Like Me!

Maybe you were just like me. In elementary school I was the uncoordinated kid. I was one of the last picked for the team. I was skinny. You get the picture. By middle and high school, I wasn't that much better. In college I started gaining weight.

I can laugh now. So much has changed. I discovered some little things that I have been doing for a long time now that seem to keep me incredibly healthy. Do you know what many of the high school jocks are doing now? They are working at a desk all day long, watching sports on the weekends, drinking a lot of beer with their friends, and getting very fat and out of shape. How do I know? I see them every day.

INTRODUCTION

What Happened to Your Body?

For the most part, we are all born with a clean slate. During the course of our lives — the day-to-day stuff, mostly — things happen that lead some of us to care for our bodies and others to neglect that important step.

That's okay. No matter what you have done to your body up until now, I honestly believe that if you decide to change today, I will be able to help you. Here's the kicker: I can't do it for you. You have to make the decision. My role is to show you and guide you through every stage and everything you need to do.

The Inside Track

For 30 plus years, I've made the commitment to better health. My doctors tell me I have the body of a 35-year-old, as opposed to my true 52 years. I would bet any amount of money that I could outrun any of the guys that were on my high school football team. If by chance any of you are reading this from Pikesville High School Class of 1972, come on... let's go! I'll prove it!

If you dream of being stronger, healthier, confident, younger-looking and more attractive to the opposite sex, you owe it to yourself to read this book. Because within these pages, I am going to teach you exactly what you need to do to turn yourself into a new person. You will discover the power of seven days. You will learn how to transform yourself into a more vibrant, healthier and physically fit YOU.

Why do some people look so good and others so terrible? I used to wonder about that. Not now. I know the answer. It took me at least 30 years to figure it out, but I can honestly say that I can teach you the answer in seven days!

To start, there is no 'theory' in this book. It's practical and has been time-tested by me. Is that good or bad? I'll let you decide. I am in the best shape of my life and it's not by accident. I can run farther than I could in high school. I can ski all day. Muscles have appeared that I never knew I had. I am thinner and stronger than I was at 30. I am 52 years old. I am loving my life.

If you dream of being stronger, healthier, confident, younger-looking and more attractive to the opposite sex, you owe it to yourself to read this book. Pay attention and find out what you can do — with my SEVEN DAY formula — to transform yourself from where you are now into a more vibrant, healthier and more physically fit you.

A Few Questions:

1. Do you feel as though you are not in your best shape?
2. Do you weigh too much?
3. Is your health questionable?
4. Do you look and feel a little older than you think you should?
5. Is your skin aging?
6. Are you tired or lazy?
7. Do you ever have a feeling that your life is OK, but could be much better?
8. Would you like people to not only notice you on the street, but also admire the way you look?

What's Going On?

We're getting older. By 2050, researchers predict that the number of Americans age 100 or older will top nearly 1 million. To get to that century-mark, doesn't it make sense to start caring for your body well in advance? Follow the secrets in this book and find out how to do it — and how to feel terrific along the way.

The fact is that with all of the resources we have, Americans are fatter and in worse physical shape than any time in history. Ten years ago, obesity in all 50 states was less than 20 percent. Today, only four states have obesity prevalence rates less than 20 percent, while 17 states had rates of more than or equal to 25 percent (Centers for Disease Control). Want more proof? Simply go to any mall, sporting event, or fast food restaurant and just look around. Go on a cruise. Pump some gas. Walk into a restaurant buffet. Observe in an airport. You will see what I mean within minutes.

I believe that given the choice, everyone would like to look young and be healthy. But many think it's impossible or out of reach to turn their lives around and look good. So they give up. Think again. I am telling you now, it is neither impossible nor out of reach to be in the best condition of your life. It can be done.

The Skinny on My Credentials

You may be wondering why you should listen to me. I am not a physician. I am a dentist by profession. I attended the University of Maryland School of Dentistry, followed by a general practice residency at East Carolina University School of Medicine in Greenville, North Carolina. I owned a very successful dental practice for 13 years.

In 1989, my brother Rich and I started The Madow Group, a company providing continuing education and specialty products for dentists. These days, the two of us spend much of our time traveling all across North America teaching dentists and their team members how to be more successful, as well as how to lead healthier lives.

It is incredible how many people flood around me to ask questions at the end of our seminars just from a brief mention that I have discovered a way for anyone to become healthier, thinner and more attractive.

My interest in exercise and health began when I learned about aerobics back in 1977. I immersed myself in the aerobics culture — reading books, running marathons, you name it. During the last 30 years, I have been experimenting with different ways to attain optimal health. What I have discovered will amaze you. I'm ready to teach you how to transform yourself. I have always had a knack for taking something that is perceived as complicated and turning it into something that is simple. It has always seemed to work for me. And that's what I am going to show you how to do right here in these chapters!

Why Listen to Me? Do I Know More Than the Other "Experts" do?

More background: Each year, I visit The Cooper Aerobics Center in Dallas, Texas for my complete physical exam. The Cooper Aerobics Center is a comprehensive health and fitness complex. Dr. Kenneth Cooper, the founder of the center, is world-renowned. I believe they are the best in the world when it comes to understanding total health.

The Center is a beautiful place, situated on 30 acres of beautifully landscaped grounds. There is a 40,000 square foot fitness center, tennis courts, a swimming pool and a jogging path that goes around the entire property. Next to the fitness center is a guest lodge where people from all over the world come to stay. And adjacent to the guest lodge is the world acclaimed Cooper Clinic, where I have the most comprehensive physical exams I have ever had in my life!

A while back during one exam, I mentioned that I was not happy with my weight and I'd like to lose about five to 10 pounds. I weighed in at about 206 pounds. The doctor felt that my weight was OK for a 6-foot-3-inch man in good physical condition. It wasn't necessary to lose weight and might be difficult to do so.

But I still wanted to be thinner. I made it my personal goal to figure out how to lose weight. To start, I was no couch potato. I was doing what I thought were all the right things: I ran, went to the gym and had a good diet. Something was just not right. I didn't want to think that losing weight would be difficult.

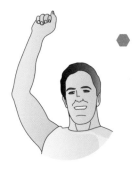

⬢ **Tell the Truth**

Are you unhappy with the way you look? Do you know in your heart you should be feeling better than you do now? Have you read a ton of exercise, diet and self-improvement books, but are more confused than ever? Take this next step.

So after a tremendous amount of experimentation, reorganization, and persistence, I figured it out! I didn't lose the five or 10 pounds that I originally wanted to lose. I lost 17 pounds! That was over 8% of my body weight! I now weigh in at a cool 189 pounds and I feel fantastic. Unlike what happens after fad diets, my weight stays the same, day in and day out.

I am 100% confident that I am in complete control of my weight. If I wanted to weigh five pounds more or five pounds less, I know I could do it. I am very happy at 189 pounds. It is the perfect weight for me. Want to know more? If you are serious about making some changes in your life, I can show you how I did it. I don't care what kind of shape you are in now. This will work for you!

I believe that after reading this book, you will put my suggestions into action. You will start seeing a difference in the way you look and feel almost immediately. I believe you will be able to get started after you read the very first chapter!

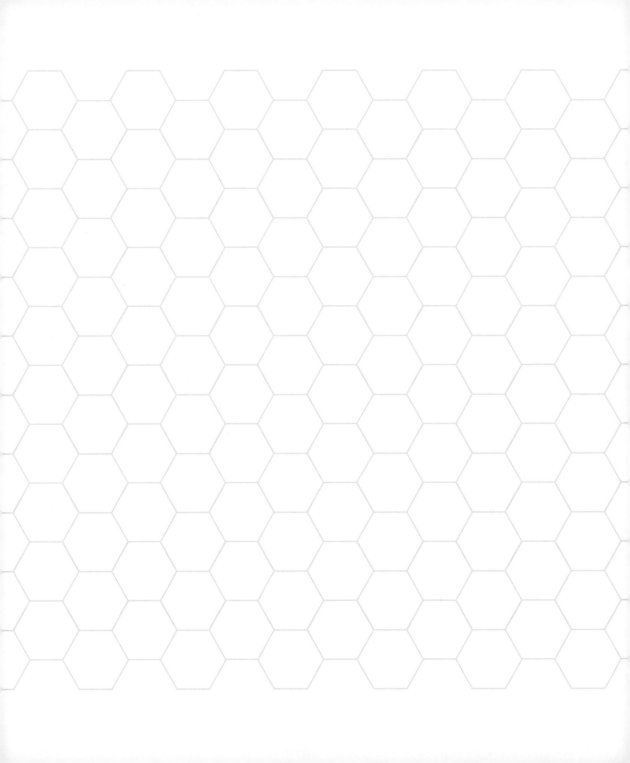

A Game Plan

This book is organized into seven chapters. Each chapter represents one day during which you can make a very real change in your life. You can take each "day" as fast or slow as you want. It's not a race.

When you finish Day Seven, you're done. You'll probably feel healthier than you ever imagined. Before you begin, it's a good idea to talk to your physician to make sure that this game plan is appropriate for your particular situation.

Are you ready to take your first step? Go to Day One.

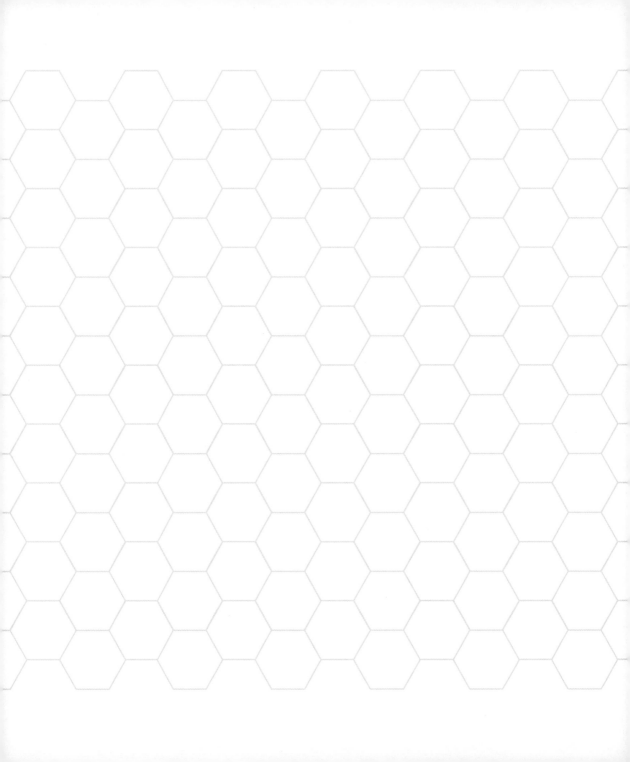

DAY ONE

Your First Decision: Change Your Life

DAY ONE

Your First Decision: Change Your Life

What would you like to do? Maybe you would like to lose some weight. Perhaps you want to get in better shape. You want to be more attractive to the opposite sex. You want to be noticed in a good way. Am I right?

⬡ Let's make a deal. Let's agree that starting today, you have made the decision to look better and feel better. Agreed?

Welcome to Day One. It's the most important of the days. Because if you don't do this, nothing else you try will work in the **end**. You may see *short-term* temporary results without Day One, but not long-lasting ones. *If you are going to put your time and energy into this, you deserve lasting results.*

If you know 'Day One,' you will be ahead of 99% of the people out there trying to get healthier and look better.

The Plan

There is no magic 'quick fix' solution. It will take time and work. If you are looking for a way to become thinner, better looking, stronger and more successful without putting in the work, this is not the plan for you.

Everything I am going to teach you, I have done and continue to do. There is no way for you to get thinner, stronger and more attractive without effort. It's impossible. So, if you pick up a book or a product that makes those claims, you are wasting your money.

I promise that I will lead you along a path that will change your life in the most positive way you could ever imagine. If you stick with me, we will get it done. You are not alone in this adventure.

Start with these words:

I have decided that
I will change my life.
In a short time
I will be thinner,
stronger, healthier,
younger looking
and more attractive.

I am ready to start!

*Decide that you are going
to change your life.
Read the message
aloud every day.*

It's a simple message. And it's a powerful message.

Here's the first step I want you to take:

⬡ **Read the message aloud every single day. That's it. You choose the time.
Never skip a day.**

Here's why it works:

⬡ **Your brain makes changes based on information that is fed to it on a regular
basis. It absolutely works! Research it more if you like. I know it works and
I am pleased to share that with you.**

One more detail:

⬡ **This exercise must be done every day. Without fail. Even as you progress
through this book, continue saying your positive Day One statement.**

Now when you are ready, let's move on to Day Two. In Day Two, you'll learn
about aerobic exercise. Aerobic means 'utilizing oxygen.' Find out why this
is important.

DAY TWO

Get Up:
Why Exercise
Rocks

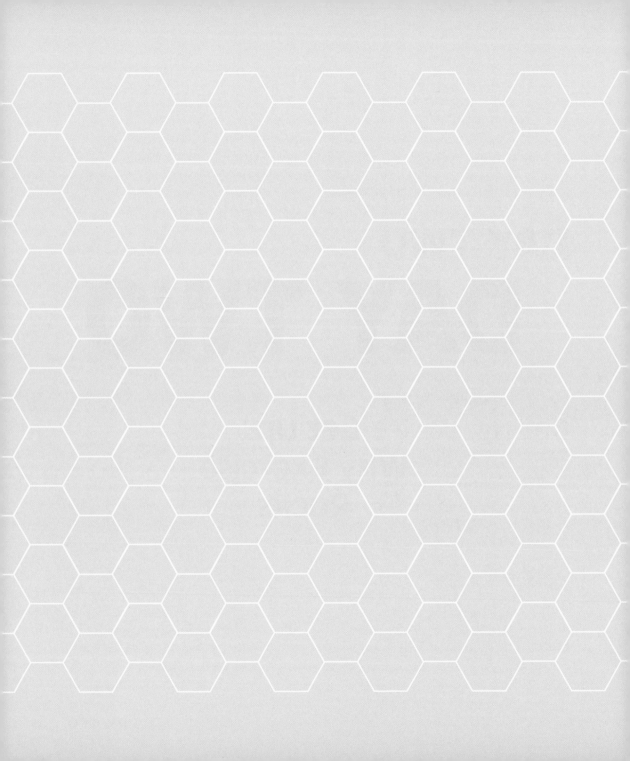

DAY TWO

Get Up: Why Exercise Rocks

How much did you move today? You're not alone if you've spent most of the day sitting on your butt. We have turned into a world of sedentary people. You drive or take public transportation to work every day. You don't do a whole lot of physical activity at school or at the office. You come home and spend time in front of the computer screen or television. Wearing a football jersey and watching sports on TV makes you feel like an athlete. You eat. You work. You go to sleep. And you get up the next day and do it all over again. Then you wonder why you are overweight. It's no wonder that heart disease is the leading killer in the United States. The American Heart Association reports that cardiovascular disease accounts for more than one-third of all deaths in the United States.

The truth though, is that exercise can be overwhelming. Who knows where to start and how much you really have to do? You're not alone. Most of the people you see exercising may be trying, but I would say that 95% of them have no idea what they are really doing. How is it benefiting them? Are they using the right muscles? Is there a better exercise that could accomplish more?

An Exercise Primer

Why does exercise have to be so complicated? Actually, it does not have to be. Truth is, there are just two types: aerobic and anaerobic.

⬡ **Aerobic = Cardiovascular (your heart and circulatory system)**

⬡ **Anaerobic = Muscles and strength (I'll talk about these exercises in Day Four.)**

Aerobic exercise uses large muscle groups continuously and is rhythmic in nature. Think of aerobics as an exercise that you can keep doing for a long period of time. The goal is to increase breathing and heart rate. Muscles are using oxygen at the same rate that you are breathing it in, creating an equal oxygen flow. Aerobic exercise is important because it conditions the heart and lungs and increases the oxygen available to the body.

⬡ **Some examples of aerobic exercise are: Running, bicycling, swimming, walking, fast dancing, rowing, and stair climbing.**

I think you get the idea.

Sedentary lifestyles increase the risk of heart attacks. The heart is a muscle with its own blood supply and it actually needs to be exercised to maintain optimum health. The best way to do that? Aerobic exercise.

What will aerobic exercise do for you?

The number one benefit is a much stronger, more efficient heart. **But it doesn't stop there!** Here are more rewards:

- Weight loss
- Improved mental health (so long, stress and depression)
- Improved immune system
- Increased stamina
- Reduction in disease
- Increased life span
- Improved muscle tone and health
- Decreased blood pressure
- Improved digestion
- Improved bone density

Begin aerobic exercise and you will start feeling healthier. Your heart muscle will become stronger, the coronary arteries will become more developed, and future exercise will require less effort.

Aerobic exercise is not difficult. It does take a commitment, though. Instead of the three times a week for 20 minutes per session that some "experts" recommend, you'll reap the most benefits if you exercise more than that.

For the exercise to be truly aerobic, you theoretically need to get your heart to beat at a certain rate for the duration of the exercise.

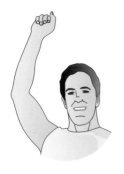

How to Calculate Your Target Heart Rate for Aerobic Exercise

Determine your maximum heart rate. Take the number 220 and subtract your age.

For an exercise to be aerobic, your heart needs to be beating between 65% and 85% of its maximum rate.

Let's say you are 40 years old. Your maximum heart rate is 220 – 40 = 180. Now if we calculate 65% of 180, we come up with 117. And if we calculate 85% of 180, we get 153.

So the zone you should be in when you exercise is between 117 and 153 heartbeats per minute.

The Best Kept Secret is Steps Away

I bike, run, swim, stair climb, and participate in road races at home and around the United States. Even so, the best exercise I've found is so simple that anyone with two healthy legs can do it just about anywhere.

It's called *walking*.

◆ **Why does walking work?**

1. You don't need special equipment. You just need a pair of comfortable shoes.

2. It's easy to begin. Just walk out your front door. You don't need to drive anywhere.

3. You can walk in most any kind of weather.

This isn't your casual stroll around the block. (Remember, I did mention that you would need to work a little.) I walk at least four miles every day on a measured course. Does that sound like a lot? It's not. And when I say every day, I mean it. Unless I have a great excuse, I'm out there. It takes me about an hour to walk my four-mile course.

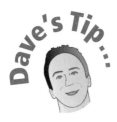

If by any chance you are a smoker, now is the time to stop. It's a dirty habit, it does not look cool, and it will kill you. Also, it's a matter of time before you will not be able to smoke anywhere in public, so why not take the steps to quit now?

Dave's Tip...

There are a million excuses about why you can't walk every day. I've heard them all. If you have a particular hurdle that could make it difficult for you to walk daily, figure out a solution. Be creative. Need advice? Email me at dave@madow.com and I'll try to help.

Here is the secret. It is not whether you walk or run, or even how far. The secret is to just get out there and do it every day. Because if you do it every day, your body will change drastically.

So what should you do right now? My answer is to start walking. Today. If you are not in your healthiest shape, you will need to start with less distance and a slower pace. That's OK. Remember, the goal is to eventually build up to the four miles and to be consistent. Better to start slowly and build your pacing.

I generally walk a mile in 14 to 15 minutes. It takes me about an hour to walk my four miles. It's a little time to spend to get great benefits. When you begin this program, start slowly with the goal of working up to four miles an hour every day. Vary your course. Weekends are a great time to push yourself a bit. Enjoy your walk. Listen to music. Your walk may become the best part of your day.

Where should you walk? Personally, I prefer outside. I have used treadmills, but I think they are boring. I like fresh air. I look at the scenery. Being outside is therapy for me. But, if the only way you can get in your walk is on a treadmill, please go for it!

Walk This Way

Although walking requires little equipment, a few things can maximize the effectiveness of your walking program.

A Shoe-in for Comfort & Support

Although you can walk in almost anything, you cannot walk distances very well in shoes that are uncomfortable and not designed for walking. Visit a store that specializes in athletic shoes, and find a knowledgeable salesperson. You need walking shoes that are supportive. It's essential that your shoes fit you right. Don't skimp.

Two-fer

Ideally, you need two identical pairs that you alternate. After a long walk, it takes some time for the cushioning to recover, so if you are using the same shoes each day, the shoes will age prematurely. Keep in mind that shoes usually need to be retired way before they look old or feel bad. Every year on my birthday, I buy two identical pairs and donate my used ones.

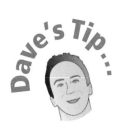

Do you absolutely have to get new shoes? My answer is no. It's more important that you get out there and walk. If you plan to walk in the shoes that you have now, please make sure they are comfortable and supportive.

Good Timing

You will need to time yourself so you don't have to guess at what pace you are walking. A runner's watch with stopwatch capability tracks your pace from beginning to end.

Best Dressed

Please wear clothes that are comfortable and appropriate for the season. In winter, wear multiple light layers, as opposed to one heavy layer. Choose clothing that breathes. Cotton gets wet and it is poor at wicking moisture away from your body. Synthetics such as polypropylene are best. For rain, a Gore-Tex outer shell layer will serve you well.

Water Works

You need water all day long. You must drink water while you walk. By the time you feel thirsty, you are already dehydrated. Don't wait until the end. I use a hip pack that holds two 16-ounce water bottles. I picked it up at the outdoor store. I drink as I'm walking. By the end of my four-mile walk, I have finished the 32 ounces.

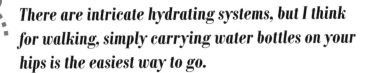

Dave's Tip... ***There are intricate hydrating systems, but I think for walking, simply carrying water bottles on your hips is the easiest way to go.***

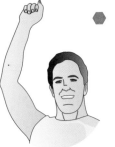

I Confess: I usually walk in the morning. But, there are days when I don't want to get out of bed. I do it anyway. When I return, I get on the scale and look in the mirror. Yes, it was definitely worth it. No question about it.

On Your Way

Aerobic exercise helps you achieve maximum health and look and feel your best. It is a lifestyle and not a fad. It is easy to find excuses why you can't do it. Make it your goal to find a way around any excuse and make sure you incorporate walking into your routine.

Please do it every day. Just find the time and do it! Your heart and body will thank you.

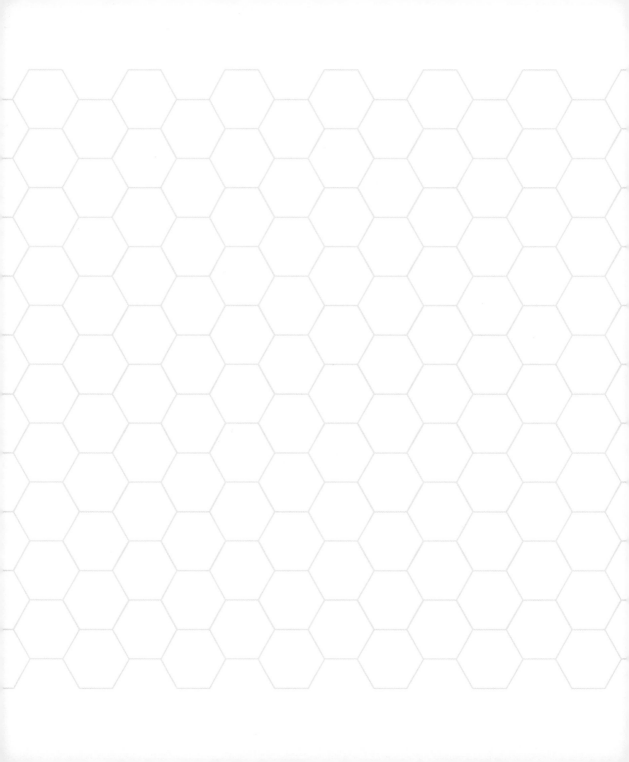

DAY THREE

Let's Eat:
My Favorite Foods Will Boost
Your Body's Potential

DAY THREE

Let's Eat: My Favorite Foods Will Boost Your Body's Potential

Did you ever stop to think what would happen if you added a solution of saturated fat, salt and sugar to the gasoline next time you filled up your car? Ugh. Imagine what it would do to the engine and other parts.

So, why do people put these products into their bodies on a daily basis and still expect their bodies to stay healthy? The foods you put into your body on a regular basis must contain nutrients that benefit cells. The reward is a healthy body that runs properly.

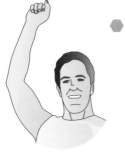

True story:

At a football game, the guy in front of me pumped so much junk into his system I wondered if he would actually show up for the next game. Here is what he ate (I took notes): A large order of French fries, popcorn, a cheeseburger, chocolate chip cookies, a large Coke and four beers. Now come on... honestly... does it sound like this gentleman will reach an old age? My bet is no.

Day Three is about putting the right food into your body. This is not about a restricted diet that makes it impossible to eat in everyday situations. It's about choosing the right foods that keep the body running in the healthiest way possible.

Here are my powerhouse foods — the ones that bring such enormous benefits to your body that they make a real difference in how you look and how you feel. These foods will transform your body into one that is healthier, more attractive, and one that will last.

There is no particular order. These foods provide extraordinary benefits.

Welcome to My Favorite Foods

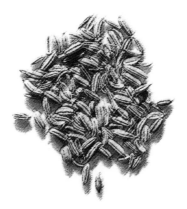

Oat Bran

Heart healthy, cholesterol reducing and easy to prepare, oat bran — the perfect breakfast food — is loaded with fiber, something we all need. Oat bran is also good for your immune system. When selecting oat bran in the grocery store, skip the instant variety. Remember, the less processed the oats are, the more fiber they will contain, maximizing the potential benefits to you. Generally the thicker the appearance of the oats, the less processed they are.

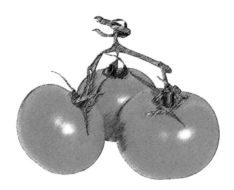

Tomatoes

Tomatoes never really made it as a "hand fruit" and that's too bad. They are loaded with so much of the anti-cancer chemical "lycopene," that I believe you should have at least one tomato every day. Lycopene is thought to protect against lung and stomach cancers and research shows that there are likely other types of cancers it may prevent. Not only that, lycopene protects you from heart attacks. Tomatoes are an excellent source of vitamin C as well. And no... drowning your burger and fries with tomato ketchup does not count. Choose the real thing.

⬡ **Attention, Men**

Harvard University researchers reported that men eating 10 servings or more weekly of tomatoes, tomato sauce or tomato juice had 45 percent fewer prostate cancers than men who ate two servings or less per week. Additionally, when men who already had prostate cancer were given lycopene supplements, they demonstrated smaller tumors, decreased malignancy rates, and less spreading of the cancer.

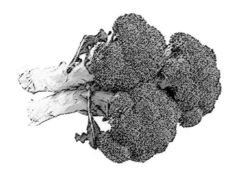

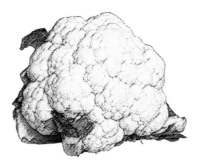

Broccoli/Cauliflower

These cruciferous vegetables are some of nature's best, most powerful health foods, containing vitamins A and C. Both are anti-cancer and anti-everything that is bad for you. The theory is that natural chemical compounds called isothiocyantes can destroy cancer cells. Try them uncooked. Eat them often. Other vegetables that are in this family are kale, cabbage and brussel sprouts. Cruciferous vegetables probably contain more cancer- fighting nutrients than any other vegetable. Broccoli and cauliflower are always at the top of my list!

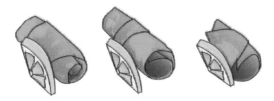

Sashimi

Sashimi is thin slices of fresh raw fish. The most common types are tuna and salmon. Both are coldwater fishes that are loaded with omega-3 fatty acids, substances that are incredibly good for your heart. Omega-3 fatty acids lower the "bad" cholesterol and make your heart feel like it's inside the body of a teenager! The oils are unique to fish. The theory is that the oils may help regulate the movement of electrolytes — calcium, potassium, and sodium, for example — through your body's cells. Besides omega-3 fatty acids, fish is full of iodine, iron and choline, which are good for the brain!

Generally, sashimi is ordered at a sushi restaurant, but Asian markets that sell fresh sashimi "ready to go" are springing up all over the place. Try to eat it a couple times weekly if possible.

If you are simply not the type to eat raw fish, some cooked tuna or salmon are fine. Also consider white-fleshed fish such as cod, flounder, halibut, orange roughy, pollack and rockfish. Although these types of fish are not as good of a source of omega-3 fatty acids, they are rich in proteins and other nutrients.

Did you know that populations that eat fish regularly live longer and have less chronic disease than populations that do not? A recent study in the *Journal of American Medicine* found that people who ate the equivalent of three ounces of salmon weekly were only half as likely to have heart disease as those who ate no fish.

Will eating a lot of fish raise my mercury level?

That is the big question. I don't have an answer. In short, we know that many types of fish do contain mercury. Mercury is a toxic substance that you do not want in your body. My feeling has always been that if you completely stay away from fish, you will miss the many nutrients mentioned above. Like anything, you must weigh the risks with the rewards.

By following these simple guidelines, I believe you can minimize your risk to mercury exposure:

1. Don't eat more than 12 ounces of most fish per week.

2. When eating canned tuna, always stick with the light tuna. Stay away or minimize the amount of albacore (white) tuna you eat.

3. Totally avoid swordfish, king mackerel, shark and tilefish. The mercury levels in these types of fish is unacceptable.

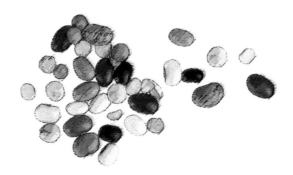

Beans

Beans contain fiber, protein and vitamins. Remember that fiber can help reduce your cholesterol levels and thus reduce your risk of heart disease. Use them in soups, cook them, or soak fresh ones overnight in water and eat them as snacks. My favorites include black beans, lentils, and garbanzos, but try them all.

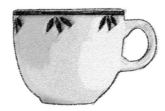

Green Tea

If there has ever been a true antioxidant "soup," this is it! I have been drinking several cups of green tea per day for at least the past 20 years. Suffice it to say there may not be another food or drink reported to have as many health benefits as green tea. The tea builds the immune system and promotes oral health, according to the UK Tea Council. Further, the drink is rich in phenolic compounds, proven to have cancer preventive effects. Drink it unsweetened.

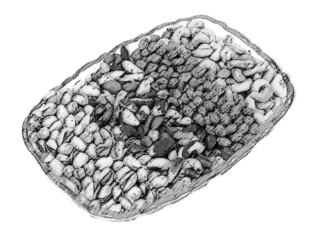

Nuts

Some people avoid nuts because of their fat content. I say "nuts" to that. Nuts are not only high in protein, but they contain the amino acid arginine, which has been shown to protect against heart disease.

The fat in nuts is mostly monounsaturated, the "good" kind of fat. That's the type of fat found in the Mediterranean diet, which has been associated with a decreased incidence of heart disease and longer life span.

Whenever I'm hungry, I grab a handful of nuts. Almonds, cashews, macadamia, and pistachios are my favorite. I love peanuts, too. While peanut butter offers benefits, choose the natural kind. The processed type is pumped full of trans-fat, which is a killer.

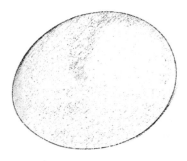

Eggs

Eggs are perhaps the best all around food. I think if I were on a desert island that had only one type of food available, I would choose the egg. Eggs are inexpensive and chock full of the highest quality protein. They contain all nine of the essential amino acids. They surpass milk, beef, whey and soy as far as protein quality.

Eggs also contain nutrients that help your eyes, brain and heart. One worth mentioning is choline, which is important in cardiovascular and brain health. Many people shy away from eggs because of their cholesterol content. That's a shame because choline helps prevent the accumulation of cholesterol and fat in the liver. I eat at least two a day. Try to get organic, from free range chickens if at all possible.

⬡ **The Yolk's On You**

I often see athletes and "health concerned people" order an egg white omelet in a restaurant. Too bad for them. The yolk has some of the most important nutrients, including choline. Please don't make the same mistake. Eat the whole egg and reap the benefits.

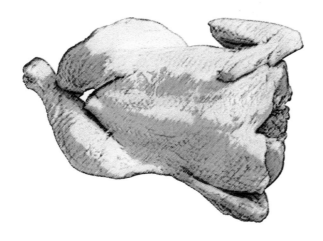

Chicken

Chicken is an excellent lean meat and a great source of high quality protein. There are also other great nutrients such as calcium, magnesium, niacin, zinc and iron. Free range, organic chickens are the best, but if you can only get the type sold at the standard grocery store, relax because the chicken still has many health benefits. One note to junk food addicts: No fried chicken or chicken nuggets. That stuff will help you get old way before your time, so stay away — unless heart disease appeals to you.

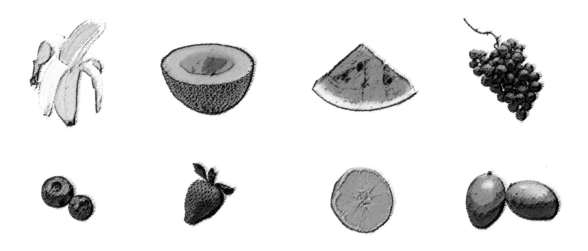

Bananas, Cantaloupe, Berries

Like vegetables, there are so many different fruits. Tops on my list are bananas, cantaloupe, watermelon, red grapes, blueberries, strawberries, oranges and mango. These are my favorites. They are loaded with fiber, anti-cancer properties, and heart-healthy vitamins. Notice the different colors; eat a rainbow of fruits and vegetables for your health.

When reviewing many of the experts "healthiest foods," there is one food that comes up on practically everyone's list. Blueberries. Blueberries are extremely rich in antioxidants and anti-inflammatory compounds that help prevent cancer and cardiovascular disease, lower cholesterol and even improve memory.

One more thing about blueberries. There is a rating system for how much antioxidant power a particular food has. It's called ORAC (oxygen radical absorbance capacity). Blueberries have one of the highest ORAC values of any food in the world.

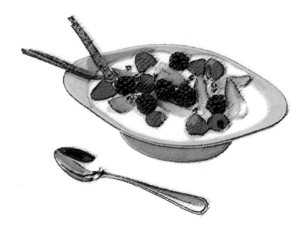

Yogurt

Plain, unsweetened yogurt is an incredibly healthy food. Sure, it contains calcium (which helps prevent osteoporosis) and protein, but that's just the beginning. Yogurt must contain active and living cultures to be yogurt. Cultures are composed of unique living microorganisms, which are responsible for many health and nutritional benefits, such as improving digestion and maximizing your body's natural defenses. Yogurt has antibacterial, antiviral and antifungal properties and is also an extremely rich source of good bacteria. Many nutritionists consider foods or supplements that aid in digestion to be extremely important to include in your diet.

Because your body is constantly waging "war" between the "bad" bugs and the "good" bugs in your digestive system, the more good bugs you throw into the equation, the less bad ones there will be. Yogurt gives you the good bugs. Of course, you can never completely get rid of the bad bugs, but you can certainly balance them out with good bacteria.

If you don't like the unsweetened type, try the vanilla, but avoid the artificially sweetened varieties.

Now That You're Eating Right... Eat Right

The Clean Plate Club has done us harm. Why do we put so much food on our plates and think that we need to eat it all?

Maybe it started when we were children and mom told us that we need to eat everything on our plate because there are starving children in China. I still have not been able to figure out how it will help the starving people if I consume everything on my plate even if I am not hungry for it. And I have yet to get a thank-you note from anyone in China acknowledging the fact that I ate everything.

To keep your weight under control, you need to take charge:

Small Meals; Very Often

I generally eat six meals each day. Surprised? Here's the difference. My meals are small. A good dinner may include some chicken vegetable soup, broccoli, and whole wheat noodles. I like to have a little something, such as some fruit, before going to bed. I often eat a little snack if I begin to feel hungry before it's time for a meal.

If you do one thing to help you with your weight and health, eating small meals should be it. It can be difficult to quantify what a 'small meal' or small portions means.

> Here's one guideline: A small meal is most likely about half of what you are eating now.

Consider a restaurant meal. When you order a steak dinner, what do you get? Chances are, you will receive a salad, an eight to 12 ounce steak (or more), a large baked potato smothered with butter and sour cream, and some vegetables. Perhaps you will order a soft drink or a beer with your meal. You'll likely have some bread before the steak is brought to the table. To finish things off, you get a piece of pie or maybe some ice cream.

What I described as a 'normal meal' is at least twice as much fat, calories and, well, food, as you should be eating. If you eat anything like this, you will gain weight. And if you are already heavy, you won't slim down.

Let's examine the meal and compare to a healthier alternative. The salad at the beginning is a good choice, as long as it's a typical dinner-sized salad and not an overflowing, oversized plate. Ask for the dressing on the side, so you can control the portion. Don't dump the dressing on the salad. Remember, the creamier the dressing, the more calories it has.

The eight- to 12-ounce steak is excessively large. The human body does not need anything larger than four ounces of meat at a meal. That is approximately the size of a deck of cards. If you want to indulge, at the very most, never eat more than six ounces.

The baked potato is fine, but only eat half if it's a big one. A sweet potato is healthier. Do not drown it in butter. Always skip the French fries or fried onion rings! They are killers. The vegetables are good as long as they are green and fresh and not soaked in butter. Ask how the food is cooked. Avoid fried foods and foods dripping in heavy sauces and butter.

Do not eat any bread. To avoid temptation, ask the waiter to take back the bread if it's on the table. No exceptions to this rule!

Skip the soft drink or beer. I never drink a soft drink, diet or otherwise. Diet drinks are unhealthy and they make you fat! Research has shown that diet drinks stimulate appetite — so you eat more when you drink diet! Alcohol is loaded with calories, so please drink in moderation. If you do drink alcohol, wine is best. Drink water — it's the best by far.

Finished your meal? Skip the dessert. You don't need the extra sugar or calories. If you crave something sweet, choose fruit.

Keep In Mind...

Eating the right foods in the right quantities is probably the most important thing you can do to achieve and maintain your proper weight. Even if you are exercising, you still need to watch what you eat. No matter how much you are exercising, it is imperative that you eat smart, too.

Eat Before You Eat

The other day, my friend and I met at a sushi restaurant. I arrived early and was hungry. So, I slipped into a nearby grocery store and bought a bag of nuts. I had a few handfuls before sitting down at the restaurant.

By doing this, I likely prevented myself from an overeating episode at the sushi place. It's so easy to overeat at a restaurant when you're hungry and with a friend. Everyone wants to eat and drink a lot when dining out. Resist the temptation. When you are hungry between meals (and you will be since you'll be eating less at each meal), eat something. Don't worry about it. Remember... you are now eating six small meals each day.

Stay Away from Dave's Worst Foods!

If you want to look good, be strong and healthy, it is imperative that you avoid certain foods that are bad for your health. These foods contribute to obesity in America. If you avoid these foods, your health will benefit.

Refined White Flour

Most bread — with the exception of some of the breads bought in a health food store — contain refined white flour, equivalent to sugar. Similarly, skip crackers and most pasta (both made with white flour). You can find pasta made of spinach or whole wheat — both far better choices.

White Rice

Eat brown rice instead. Brown rice is essentially white rice that has not had the nutritious bran covering removed. A cup of brown rice has 3.5 grams of fiber, versus a cup of white rice that has less than one gram of fiber. The bran also contains nutrients such as magnesium, manganese and zinc.

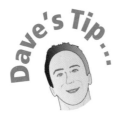

A rough rule of thumb to go by when eating is 'don't eat anything white.' Two exceptions are cauliflower and white fish.

Highly Processed Foods

If it's made in a lab and has ingredients that you can't pronounce, please don't put it in your body!

Sugar is Not Sweet

Americans today eat 30 times more sugar than our ancestors did 200 years ago. High sugar is linked to tooth decay and obesity, as well as myriad of other diseases. For your health, reduce your sugar intake drastically. Or better yet, avoid it. One of the biggest problems is that sugar is hidden in a high percentage of the foods that you are eating right now.

Read labels on all food before you buy it. If you see any of the following ingredients listed — don't bring that product home.

High Fructose Corn Syrup

This is a corn starch product that is manufactured into a thick liquid containing equal parts fructose and sucrose — both sugars. Research is just beginning to show that high fructose corn syrup may be treated more like a fat in the body, skewing the hormones responsible for weight management.

⬡ Is it Real?

While in an airport, I was craving a fruit drink and I saw a smoothie advertised at a fast food restaurant. The description read bananas, strawberries and kiwi blended with 10 types of fruit juice. It sounded very healthy. I was just about to order one when I asked about the kind of fruit juice they use. The server held up a huge jug of "juice." When I looked at the ingredients, the first one ingredient was "high fructose corn syrup," another word for concentrated sugar. Ugh. I said "thanks" and then simply walked away.

Sugar Free Has a Price

I see so many people consuming drinks and foods that are "sugar free" but contain artificial sweeteners. As bad as refined sugar is, these chemicals are a million times worse. If you are drinking diet sodas to stay slim, stop immediately!

It's not only because artificial sweeteners are poison. That's just part of the story. They will also make you fat. Drink one of those "diets," and you will gain weight!

Here's why: When we eat sugar, the pancreas secretes insulin. Insulin is a hormone that is responsible for regulating the amount of sugar circulating in your blood. Insulin attaches to the sugar, and carries it off into the cells.

Now look at what happens when you ingest an artificial sweetener. Your body senses something sweet and it believes it's sugar. Since your blood sugar regulating mechanism does not distinguish between "real" sugar and artificial sugar, the pancreas secretes insulin to balance out the sugar in the blood. But there is no sugar to attach to the insulin.

Because our body doesn't just like to have free insulin floating around, it desperately needs to find some sugar. How does it do this? Your body says "I'm hungry." And you eat. Voila! Now there is something to bind with the insulin. It happens every time. And this makes you fat.

Diet drinks and artificial sweeteners. Your best bet? Stay away.

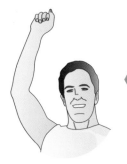

I confess: It's so tempting to eat foods that are not particularly healthy. If you need one rule to live by, please make it the one that I live by — **never eat sweets**.

Trans Fat

Trans fat lowers your HDL cholesterol (the good one) and raises your LDL cholesterol (the bad one). Low HDL and high LDL is a risk factor for heart disease. Commercial baked goods — such as crackers, cookies and cakes — and many fried foods such as doughnuts and French fries — contain trans fat. Shortenings and some margarines also are high in trans fat. Avoid trans fat all costs, it will kill you!

Artificial Sweeteners

These sweetener go by many names: saccharin, aspartame, acesulfame, potassium sucrolase, neotame cyclamate. If you can't pronounce it, don't eat it. If you can pronounce it, don't eat it either!

Soft Drinks

You don't need the sugar or chemicals. There is nothing in the drinks that help you stay healthy. Sodas offer no nutritional value. Drink fresh water.

So there you have it... the top foods that will keep you healthy and young, as well as the foods and ingredients you will need to avoid. With this in mind, it's time to move to Day Four.

DAY FOUR

Pump It Up:
It's Time to Get Stronger!

DAY FOUR

Pump It Up:
It's Time to Get Stronger!

So far, we have learned about how important aerobic exercise is, as well as eating the right foods. On Day Four, it's time to tackle another type of exercise — you probably know it as weight training.

Weight training is moving your muscles against resistance. This is done by pushing or pulling weights. As contrasted with running and walking, weight or strength training is *anaerobic*, meaning the muscles are exercised at a high intensity for a short period of time. Anaerobic means "without oxygen," and that's why this type of exercise can only be performed in short "bursts." Besides lifting weights, sprinting is another example of anaerobic exercise.

Beyond Running and Walking

Even though I was doing aerobic exercise for 25 years, I kept thinking that I was missing something. I didn't see how I could properly exercise all of the muscles in my body. So about four years ago, I took action. I called a personal trainer.

At the first appointment, we worked for a full hour and I learned exercises to strengthen my chest, shoulder, and abdominal muscles. Later, I would learn how to address my leg muscles, and then back and arm muscles.

During anaerobic exercise, the muscles are using oxygen at a higher rate than you are breathing it in, creating a 'negative' oxygen flow. Lactic acid is the byproduct that builds up in your muscles during anaerobic exercise. When oxygen is limited, lactate allows glucose to breakdown and energy production to continue.

There are different anaerobic exercises (just think of all of the different muscles you have). Hiring a personal trainer is a great way to learn how to perform the exercises correctly. If you do not perform them correctly and efficiently, you risk injury.

The benefits of strength training are incredible:

- increased strength
- increased confidence
- maintaining lean body mass
- decreased risk of osteoporosis
- preventing injuries resulting from weak muscles
- better balance/posture
- increased metabolism (you burn more calories 24 hours a day!)
- increased energy
- improved immune system
- improved mental health

Age is not a barrier to weight training. An elderly debilitated woman with rheumatoid arthritis came into my trainer's gym asking for help. She could hardly walk to the door of the gym. Over time, through strength training, he was able to help her become stronger and actually reverse some of the effects of the arthritis.

Do you think he had her lifting 30-pound weights? Of course not! She began by lifting a small soup can in each hand. By the time she left his program, she was stronger, walked with much better posture, felt younger, had more confidence, and was able to do many things she thought she'd never be able to do again in her life.

There is no question in my mind that training with weights has made me feel better than I have in my entire life. It is one of the best things you can do for your body. It is so important that it needs to be part of your regimen.

Can you exercise on your own? As I said earlier, a trainer would be a great way to get started. But if joining a gym or hiring one is not possible, please don't worry. I am going to show you some very basic strength exercises that you can do by yourself in the privacy of your home.

C'mon In

I know many of you are afraid to walk into a gym and are intimidated about it. I was the same way. I thought all the muscle men would laugh at me. They would wonder what someone like me was doing in 'their' gym.

I was wrong. Because of my travel schedule, I have visited many gyms all over the United States, as well as internationally. The people I have met are some of the nicest people, with no hidden agendas, no egos and a true willingness to help me if I had any questions. If you are thinking about working out at gym, try it. You'll find a supportive group of people.

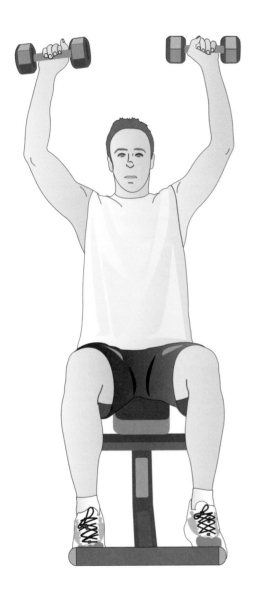

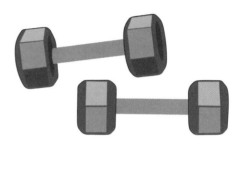

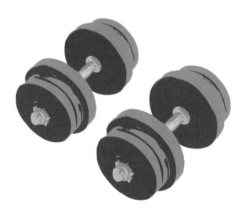

Step One:

Visit your local sporting goods store and buy a pair of dumbbells. Dumbbells are free weights that are designed to be held in your hands.

Dumbbells come in different weights. The best thing to do would be to have several pairs in your collection.

⬡ **If you are female: Start with dumbbells weighing two, five and eight pounds. This is just a guideline and you may choose weights depending on your strength and weight.**

⬡ **If you are male: Start with dumbbells weighing five, 10 and 15 pounds. Again, this will vary depending on your strength and weight.**

Although dumbbells are most commonly a solid fixed weight, you may want to look for the type of dumbbells that are adjustable, meaning you can make them heavier or lighter simply by adding or removing the weights that come with them. This may be the best idea because you probably won't be able to tell what weight or weights will work best until you actually start using them.

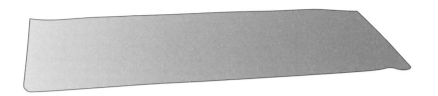

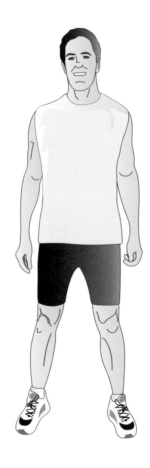

Impress the World with Your Body in Seven Days

Step Two:

It's helpful to have a comfortable mat to lie on while performing these exercises. Find one at the same store where you purchase your dumbbells. You will also need a basic chair to perform some of the exercises.

Step Three:

Wear the right clothes. Skip the expensive exercise clothes while performing strength exercises. Choose clothing that is comfortable and gives you complete freedom of movement.

A tee-shirt or a sleeveless muscle shirt is a good choice. Select a wickable, breathable material, instead of cotton, which will retain moisture instead of getting rid of it (wicking it away). Running shorts or bicycle shorts work well. Again, no cotton.

Wear tennis shoes, sneakers, running or walking shoes. Be sure to wear socks to help absorb sweat. If you ever exercise without socks, you set yourself up for foot infections due to the warm, moist environment you are creating.

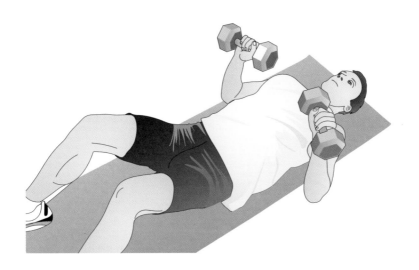

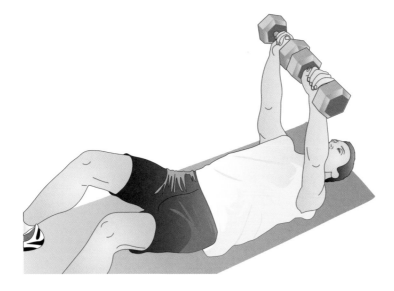

Great Exercises

Here are some great basic strength exercises that you should be able to perform easily at home or in the gym. Read through them first just for a basic understanding. Feel free to refer back to these pages while exercising to ensure you are doing them correctly. At the end of Day Four I will let you know how often you should be doing these exercises.

Please understand that the exercises I describe below are basic and not meant to be all encompassing. The goal is not to turn you into a bodybuilder. We want to strengthen major muscle groups. If at any time you want to take it to the next level, there are plenty of books and videos out there that will help you.

Chest Press

Start by lying face up on your mat. Take a dumbbell in each hand and hold them against your chest (position 1).

Now extend your arms straight up into the air and touch the dumbbells together at the top (position 2). Bring your arms back down to position 1. This is considered one full repetition (rep). Do eight reps. Eight reps is one set. Rest for 30 seconds and repeat another eight reps. Rest for 30 seconds and repeat one more time.

As with all of the exercises I am teaching you, if you find them too difficult, you will need to use lighter dumbbells. If it's way too easy for you and it doesn't feel as though you are doing anything at all, use slightly heavier dumbbells.

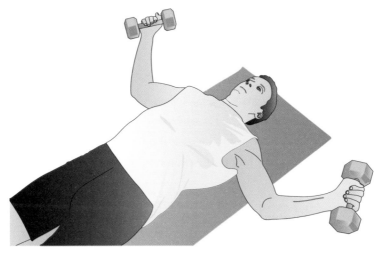

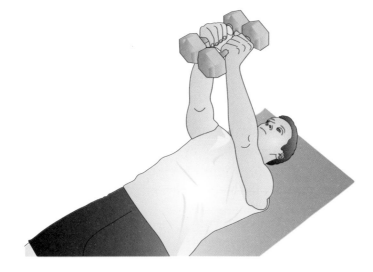

Impress the World with Your Body in Seven Days

Flat Fly (Chest)

While lying on the mat, take a dumbbell in each hand and place each by your side (position 1). Now pretend there is a large object suspended in the air just above your body. Your objective is to bring the weights up and wrap them around the object without touching it and ultimately get the weights to come together in the very top position (position 2). Then, bring the weights back down to the starting position (position 1). You have just completed one rep. Do three sets of eight reps with a thirty-second rest between each set. And if the exercise is way too easy or difficult, please adjust the weight of the dumbbells.

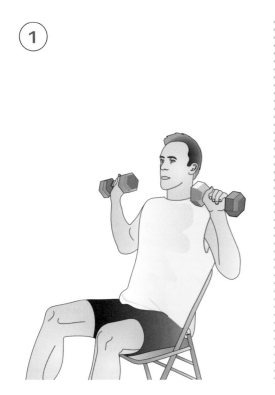

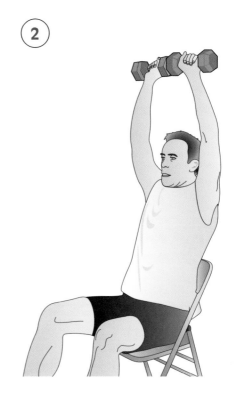

Shoulder Press

This exercise is similar to the chest press, but is performed sitting in a chair. Start with a dumbbell in each hand with your arms up parallel to the wall (position 1). Raise each arm to the ceiling and touch the dumbbells together at the highest position (position 2). Now bring them back to position 1. Do a total of three sets of eight reps, with about thirty seconds of rest in between each set.

Again, if the exercise is too easy or difficult, adjust the weight of the dumbbells.

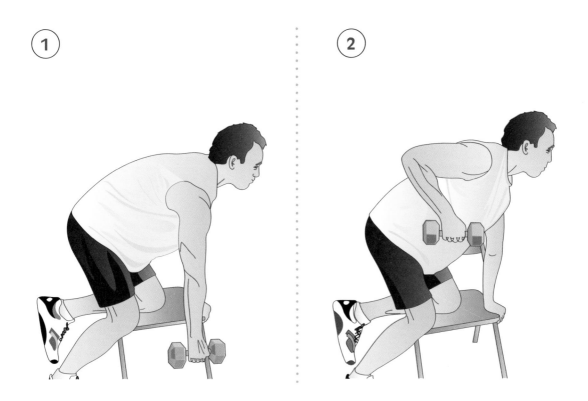

One Arm Row (Back Muscles)

Use a chair with a padded seat. Take one dumbbell in your right hand. Bend your left leg and rest it on the chair, while letting the dumbbell hang freely from your right hand as shown in position 1. Slowly raise the dumbbell up to the right side of your chest as shown in position 2. Now lower it down to position 1 again. This is one rep. Do eight of these reps.

Transfer the dumbbell to your left hand and place your right leg on the chair. Do eight reps in this position. You have now completed one full set. Do a total of three sets.

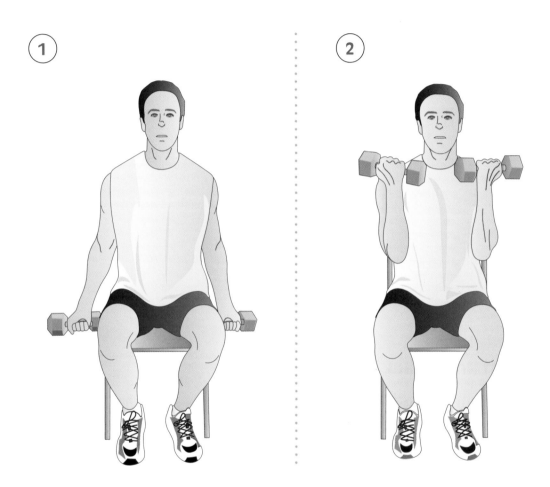

Curl (Biceps)

Sit on the edge of a chair with one dumbbell in each of your hands. Let your hands drop freely so they are in front of you facing outward with the dumbbells in place. This is starting position 1. Bring the dumbbells toward your chest by only bending your elbows. Do not turn your arms or wrists. You are in position 2. Straighten your elbows and return to starting position 1. This is one rep. Do three sets of eight reps.

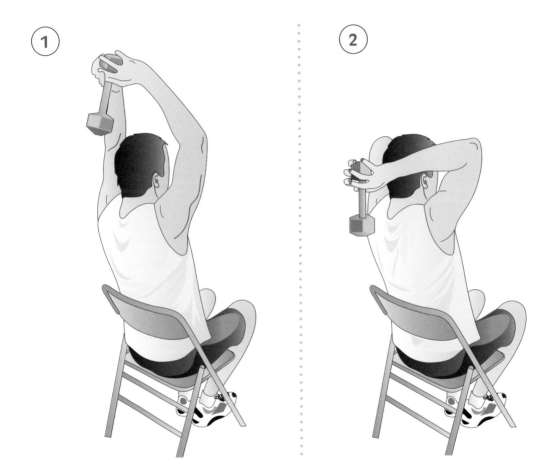

Double Arm Pullover (Triceps)

Sit down in a chair. Lift a single dumbbell over your head with both hands. This is position 1. Gently lower the dumbbell behind your back. While doing this, please try to keep your elbows as close to your body as possible. This is position 2. Now come back up to position 1. You have now completed one rep. Do three sets of eight reps each.

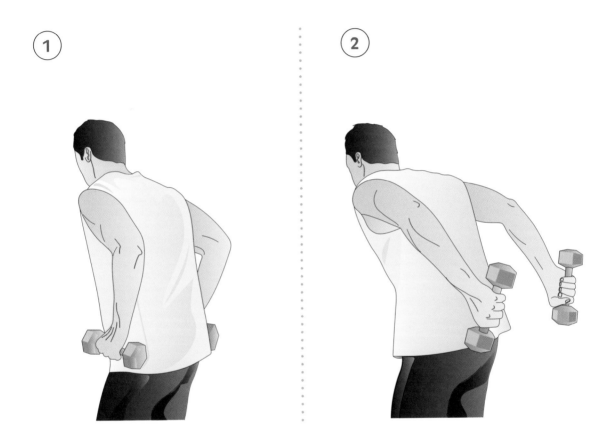

Impress the World with Your Body in Seven Days

Double Arm Kickbacks (Triceps)

Stand up and take a dumbbell in each hand and place them in the starting position 1. Now while keeping your elbows tucked in close to your sides, simultaneously slowly raise each weight to position 2. Slowly move the weights back to the starting position. This is one rep. Try doing two sets of ten reps each. It is very important to keep your elbows tucked in and not to swing your arms. Otherwise, you will get no benefit from this exercise!

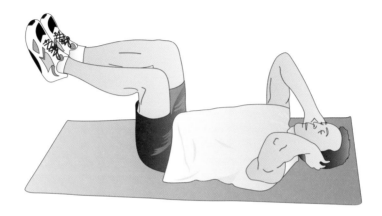

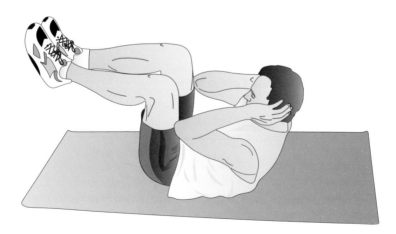

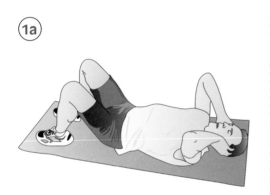

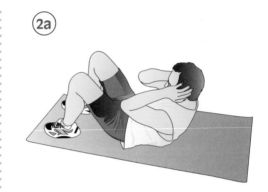

Crunches (Abdominal Muscles)

Lay flat on your mat facing up. Bring your knees in close to you and keep them bent so your legs will remain parallel to the floor. This is position 1. Bring your head forward a little as you gently raise your upper body slightly off the ground. This is position 2. Do not come up all the way or you are not doing a crunch anymore – you're doing a sit-up! Come back down into position 1. That is one rep. Let's do three sets of eight reps each of these crunches.

An alternate to position 1 would be to bend your knees while keeping your feet flat on the ground (positions 1a & 2a).

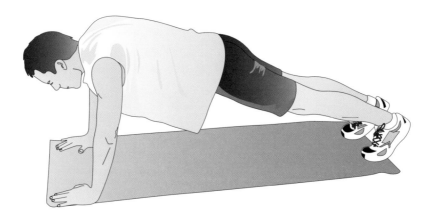

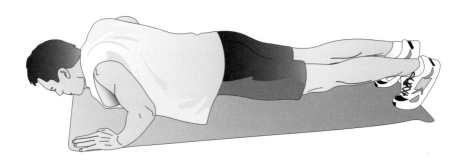

Impress the World with Your Body in Seven Days

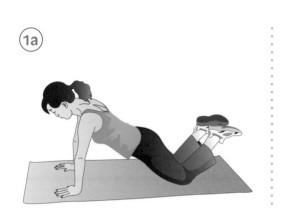

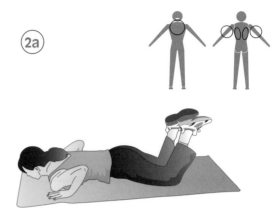

Push-ups (Perhaps the best all around exercise!)

Support yourself with your hands on the mat as seen in position 1. Keep your body as straight as possible. The only things touching the mat should be the balls of your feet and your hands. Now, keeping your body straight, lower yourself down until your face almost touches the floor. You are now in position 2. Slowly push yourself back into position 1 and you have completed one full rep.

If you are not able to maintain this position, you may do a variance of this exercise on your knees instead of your feet as seen in position 1a. Now, keeping your body straight, lower yourself down until your face almost touches the floor. You are now in position 2a if you are doing the alternate version. Slowly push yourself back into position 1a and you have completed one full rep.

⬡ If you are not used to doing push-ups, it may be very difficult to do eight reps. At first, you do as many as you can comfortably do. Whatever that number is, please do three sets. Then over time, work your way up to doing three sets of eight reps. If you are doing the alternate version, ultimately try to change over to the standard pushup when you can.

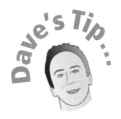

⬤ Keep in mind that it is possible to injure yourself if you start too fast and use too much weight. Err on the side of too little weight, and then increase when you can. The object of strength exercises is to start slowly and build up strength.

How Often?

How frequently should you do the nine strength exercises? Start once per week. Combined with everything else that you will be doing, that is plenty. After time, if you are super motivated and want more, you may do these twice a week, but I would not recommend any more than that in order to give your muscles the proper recovery time.

Also, please understand that muscle has great memory and adapts to exercise. Eventually, if you continue using the same weights, you will see less results. As you progress, increase the weight or the number of reps you do at one time. The best approach is to increase both weight and number of reps.

If you are thinking about guidance with any of the "days" in this book, hiring a personal trainer at the local gym or fitness center would definitely be of value with Day Four!

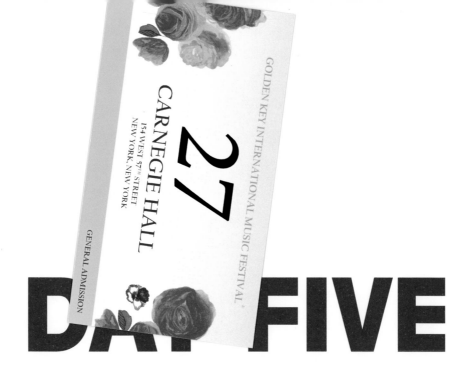

DAY FIVE

Stretch:
That Feels Good

DAY FIVE

Stretch: That Feels Good

When it comes to doing important things for your body, stretching is vital. It's also forgotten a great deal of the time. Either we don't know how, we don't have time or we think it's unimportant. The result? We suffer from aches and pains that cannot be explained. Many of you visit your physician, chiropractor, podiatrist, acupuncturist, and physical therapist for problems that could very likely be addressed with daily stretching.

Why Do We Need to Stretch?

During the course of the day, your muscles tighten from normal activity. If you exercise, they become tighter. Even when you sleep, your muscles tighten. And when muscles tighten, they tend to pull your body parts to places where they shouldn't be. Taking a few minutes each day to stretch will make you feel like a new person.

Here are some basic stretches that lead to great results.

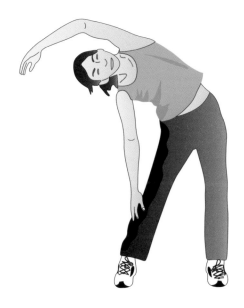

Side Stretch

Stand straight and raise your left arm over your head while keeping your right arm by your side. Slowly bring your left arm over to the right as far as you can while bending to the right at your waist. Hold for 20 seconds. Now return to start and repeat this two more times. Repeat this stretch three times on the opposite side.

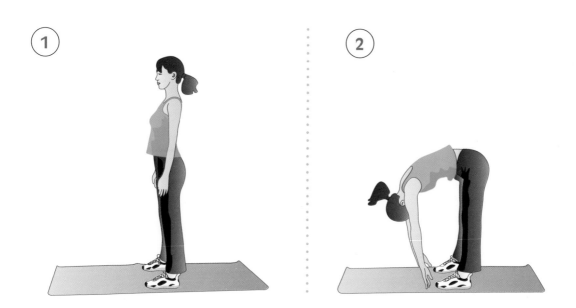

Toe Touches

Toe touches stretch out the hamstring muscles of the back of your upper leg. Tight hamstrings cause lower back pain. Begin by standing up straight (position 1). Without bending your knees, slowly reach down and touch your toes with your fingers, as far as you can (position 2). It doesn't matter if you can go all the way down. Just go as far as you can. Hold the position for 20 seconds and return to the starting position. Do this three times!

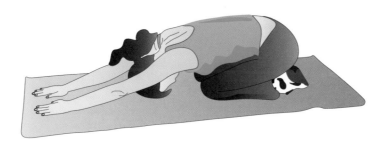

Child's Pose

This fantastic exercise keeps your back in great shape. Place your mat on the floor and sit down on your knees. Keeping your arms over your head, slowly lower your upper body until your face is against the mat. Hold this stretch for 20 seconds. Relax and rest for about 30 seconds. Repeat for a total of three stretches.

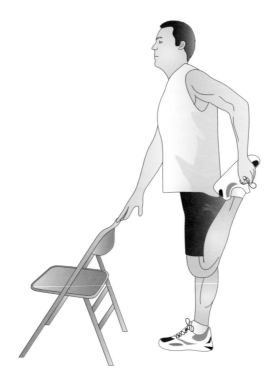

Quads Stretch

Stand up facing a wall and bend your right leg at the knee as far back as you can. Support yourself against the wall with your left hand. Using your right hand, keep as much pressure as possible on your right leg so that you feel the stretch in your right quads (the large muscle in the front upper part of your leg). Hold this stretch for 20 seconds and release. Repeat for the left leg. Continue until you have performed this stretch three times on each leg.

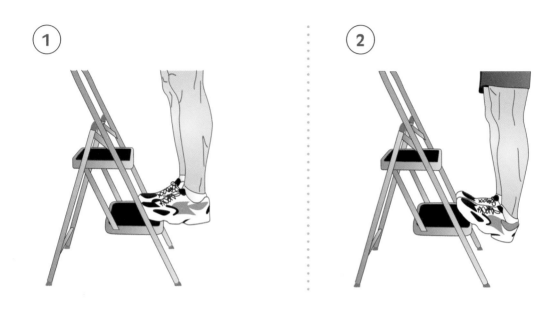

Calf Stretch

Stand on the edge of a step or a ledge, touching with only the front third of your feet (position 1). Keeping strong contact with the step, lower the back of your feet until you feel a strong stretch in the calf muscles in the back of your lower leg. This is position 2. Hold the stretch for 20 seconds and then return to position 1. Repeat for three stretches.

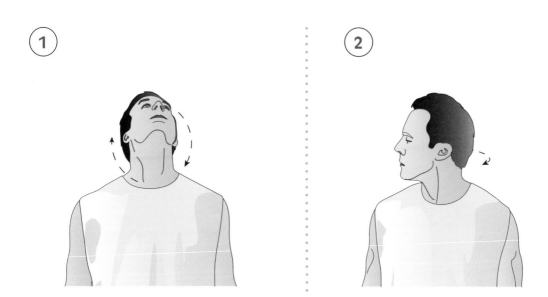

Neck Stretch

Look forward and rotate your head slowly in a clockwise direction. It's easy to do this if you just think of your nose as the central point that is drawing a circle in the air. Do this for about twenty seconds and then reverse the direction. This will loosen up the neck muscles (motion 1).

Looking straight ahead, turn your head all the way to the right as far as you can. (motion 2) Hold 20 seconds. Now turn to the left and hold 20 seconds. Repeat for a total of three times.

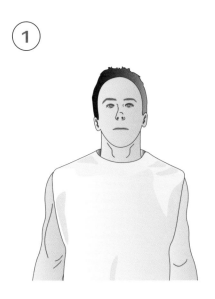

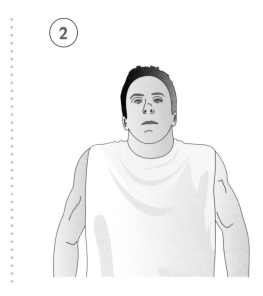

Shoulder Stretch

Stand up and look straight ahead (position 1). Shrug your shoulders and hold them in that position for 20 seconds. Release and relax. Repeat this stretch for a total of three times (position 2).

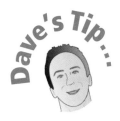

Dave's Tip...

If you take the time to do some daily stretching, you can avoid much, if not all, of the pain and ailments that people develop over time from not doing so!

Try to stretch every day. As with the strength exercises in Day Four, the stretches in Day Five are not meant to be all inclusive. There are definitely many more stretches you can do. But the ones I have described here are great basic stretches that are an integral part of the 'Seven Days.' There is no question in my mind that they will make you feel fantastic.

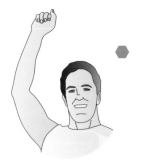

I confess: Sometimes I forget to stretch. When I do, my body has a funny way of reminding me by tightening up all of my muscles. Then I remember how important my stretching routine is.

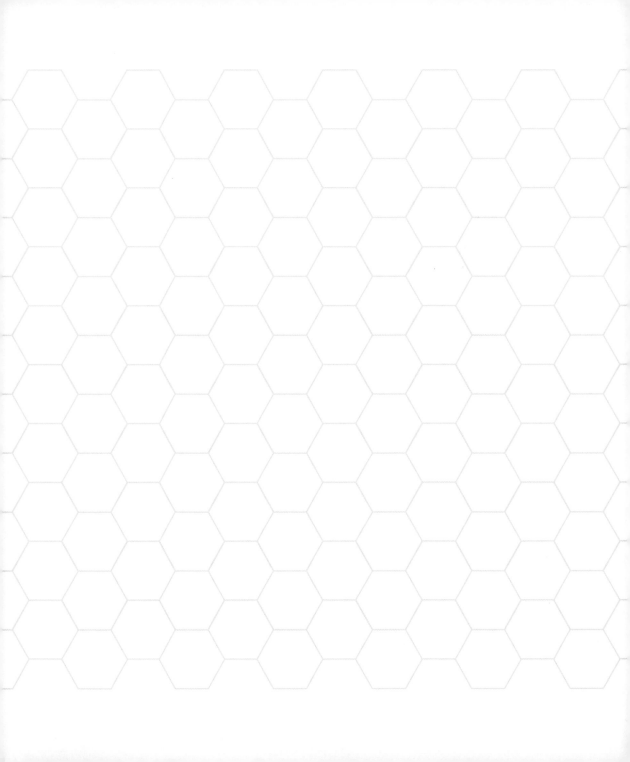

DAY SIX

Drink Water:
Be a Regular Person!

DAY SIX

Drink Water: Be a Regular Person!

Our bodies are made up of about 65 percent water. Every minute, our bodily functions are causing us to lose water. That lost water must be replenished. It takes an average of eight to 10 cups of water (above and beyond the water that we get in our food) to replenish what our bodies lose each day. Most of us are dehydrated, but we don't know it because we aren't thirsty.

When we don't drink water, our bodies suffer. The solution? Drink eight glasses of pure fresh water every day. Since the average glass of water is eight ounces, this will come to a total of 64 ounces daily. Sounds like a lot of water? If you spread it out during the the day, it's easier to do.

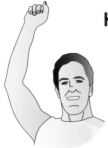

Here are the benefits of drinking water:

- Your skin and hair start looking better.
- Your joints become more lubricated.
- You digest your food better.
- You eliminate waste more regularly.

The Scoop on Water

Water is the only drink that keeps you properly hydrated. You have to drink it. Water does not mean soda, tea, coffee, alcohol or juice.

About 10 years ago, I realized how water, exercise and food make the body function. During a trip to the Grand Canyon, a friend and I went on a three-day backpacking trip deep into the inner canyon. We carried the supplies on our backs and walked difficult terrain for three days. It was hot. Other than walking, the main activities were eating and drinking. We had to eat and drink all day to stay strong enough to walk.

Contrast that to my sedentary days. When I sat in my office all day long, I would snack on junk that wasn't good for me. I never thought about drinking water. Since my body was not moving much at all, my bodily functions were much slower. I felt OK, but not 100%. Was this healthy? Was it natural?

When I was backpacking in the Grand Canyon, I was forced to eat and drink healthy all day long. The combination of exercise, eating and drinking made me feel fantastic. I started noticing more about my body.

Regular... Means Regular

One of the first changes had to do with the bathroom. I began having more daily bowel movements than ever before. I went to the bathroom about three times a day. I finally found out how good it felt to eliminate waste from my body the way nature intended. I realized firsthand the role of water in the intestines and its important function in passing waste material through the body.

I cringe when I hear physicians say it is normal for some people to have a bowel movement once every two days. That is really saying that a lot of waste material is moving very slowly or is stuck somewhere in the confines of the intestine. It's a formula for gas, bloating, toxicity and disease. That doesn't sound so normal to me.

Think about infants and their bodily functions. When babies are fed, they have a bowel movement. This is normal and the way nature intended. As babies get older, they learn to wait, or hold in, their bowel movement. Add to that a diet that is low in fiber, physical inactivity, and not enough water, and this becomes the recipe for constipation and fecal impactions.

It has been said that many people are walking around with large amounts of impactions in their gut. It is not uncommon for an adult to carry five to 10 pounds of impacted fecal material. That is heavy, not to mention toxic.

Are you constipated right now or have you had some problems with constipation in the past? Most likely you have fecal material that is lodged somewhere in the recesses of your large intestine. Chances are, it's been there for a long time. It's toxic, unhealthy and dangerous.

When I was sedentary, I had many bouts with constipation and irregularity. I figured it was normal to go a day or two without having a bowel movement. I was sure that the bloating and the gas were perfectly fine as well.

Never again! I am eliminating the toxins from my body every day like clockwork. I practically guarantee that if you follow my seven-day plan, you will see an amazing difference in how you eliminate your waste products and how much better you feel.

Would you rather get the waste out of your body as often as possible or would you prefer to keep it in? Drink water. One of the easiest ways to keep track of how much water you are drinking is to carry a refillable water bottle around with you. I use a 32-ounce Nalgene bottle and carry it with me to the office and when I go out. Drink your water every day.

People ask me whether I drink tap or bottled water. I mostly drink bottled spring water from a reputable vendor. There are impurities in tap water. The amount and type of impurities vary from area to area. Since I travel so much, I want to be safe. Sure, bottled water is expensive. I look at it as insurance. It is worth it to my body to ingest the purest food and drink available. That is not to say I never drink from the tap. I do, but if given the choice, I will always choose bottled spring water.

Dave's Tip...

Drink water throughout the day. When you finish eight glasses (64 ounces) of fresh water, you're done.

Why Water?

Suppose you are hiking in the mountains. You thought you brought enough water, but halfway through the hike, you notice you are running dangerously low. If you don't find some type of a natural water source soon, you risk serious dehydration. And you know that dehydration will lead to death!

Suddenly, you come across water. Even better, it's your lucky day because you find two different sources!

The first source is a freshwater stream running across rocks. It's clean and clear. The second source is not as pretty. It's a small pond filled with green, algae-laden water with a thick film of surface scum. Mosquitoes are buzzing.

Which one do you want to drink? The clean, flowing water or the dirty scummy water? Seems like a no-brainer to me!

Let's apply this analogy to the water in your body. (Remember, it makes up about 65 percent). Would you rather replenish the water frequently so it is fresh (think clean stream) or not replenish it enough so it resembles the scummy pond?

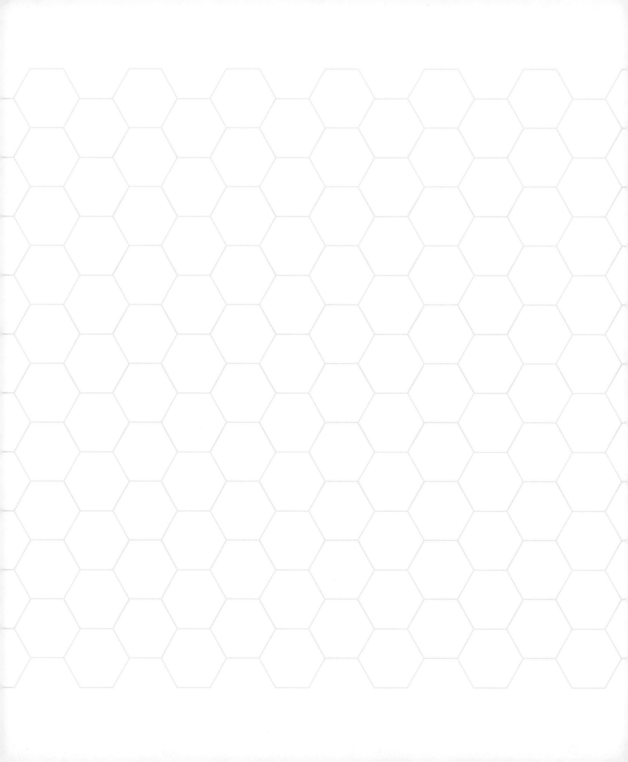

DAY SEVEN

Putting It Together:
The Most Important Day

DAY SEVEN

Putting It Together: The Most Important Day

Until now, the game plan has been concrete: exercise and eating. The most important concept to remember is that it's not about reading the words on the page — it's about putting the words into action. You need to do something to transform your body into something you probably never dreamed you could. *You can do this.*

Welcome to Day Seven. Today has a different spin. It's not as defined the same way as the earlier days. I think it's the most difficult day to master. Here's the best part: Once you do achieve these goals, your body will achieve a fitness level you probably never imagined.

What's Going On?

We've talked about your physical self — what you put into your body and what you do to your body. Now, it's time to talk about another factor affecting your physical health — your emotional self.

We need to be at peace with ourselves and with others. A mind and a body that are in a state of harmony will lead to a long, healthy life. Disease and early aging are not normal. They are caused by something going awry in your cells.

I believe that the mind plays an enormous role in what happens to us physically. Stress is a killer. Even if you are doing everything right concerning exercise and diet, when you are not at ease, your body's cells are under attack. The damage may not show up for years, but it is taking place quietly. One day it just may rear its ugly little head in the form of some type of disease.

So the big question: How can you tell if your mental condition is OK? The answer is... most likely, you know deep down inside if you have a total feeling of peace. The reason I say "deep down" is that many people have a lot going on beneath the surface, but choose to pretend that everything is fine. Some can hide feelings so deep, that they almost forget they are there. And no matter how much you try to hide and act, negative feelings may be festering inside and doing serious damage.

- Are you happy?
- Do you enjoy your life?
- Are you stressed?
- Are you sad? Nervous? Moody?
- Do you fight with people easily?
- Do you find it hard to forgive someone?
- Do you laugh often?
- Do you smoke?
- Do you use alcohol or drugs to feel better?
- If there is anything you'd like to do differently, what would it be?

Take a Drive

Want to know more? Start with "Dave's Driving Test." Next time you are driving to your workplace, take a step back and reflect. Be totally honest with yourself. How do you feel? Are you happy to be going to work? Do you look forward to your job? Are you excited? Or are you thinking, "Another day at work, I can't wait until five o'clock."

You don't have to be driving. You could be walking or on public transportation. But it is very important to see how you feel while you are on your way. If you are not truly excited to be going to your job, you need to reevaluate what you are doing. You most likely spend many hours each week working. Dreading what you do for a living will eat away at your body.

The next morning while going to work, think about other stressors in your life. Could it be money? A relationship? Family? A problem with a friend? Something you have not been honest about with yourself or others? Zero in on the problem and determine why this is causing stress in your life.

If you find things in your life that are getting in the way of achieving peace of mind, then you MUST determine a way to get rid of them. It is not an option to live with something that is standing in the way of a peaceful mind. It may ultimately cause disease.

I believe there is an answer to every problem. It may take the assistance of a counselor therapist to help you, but I cannot overemphasize how important it is to get rid of the bad stuff in your life.

Day Seven is Not Simple.

It's not easy. It's not a matter of one-two-three. It will make you look at yourself in a way that you may never have looked at yourself before. If you are honest with yourself and take care of the troublesome areas of your life, you will achieve peace and health that will help you complete the Seven Days.

THE WEEK IS OVER

Now What?

You now know what it takes to "Impress the World With Your Body in Seven Days." Congratulations! But will simply reading this book guarantee your success? Absolutely not.

It's far too easy to read the book, agree with its content … and then put it back on the shelf. You can do better. Promise yourself that you will follow these techniques. Promise yourself that you will change your activity level, eat better, walk more, drink more water and care for yourself inside and out.

You can follow through. Because I know you truly would like to be healthier, stronger and more attractive to the opposite sex. You know you can.

Dave's Tip…

Take two good pictures of yourself today. One should be your full body and the other a head shot. Then take two pictures in the same poses on the first day of each month. Keep the pictures in order in a nice photo album. My bet is that in a very short time you will love what you see. Good Luck!

Dave

MORE IDEAS TO GET YOU GOING

Ten Tips to Continued Success

1 Be Careful with Antibiotics

It seems that antibiotics are prescribed as if they were candy. Pretty soon they'll be sold alongside beer and popcorn at sporting events. Whether for an illness or dental procedure, you'll receive an antibiotic. We're so used to the regimen that we never stop to think of the ramifications of taking antibiotics.

The word antibiotic means against life. When you take an antibiotic, it not only goes after the bad bacteria, but it begins killing off the good ones as well. Take antibiotics and you may wipe out the good bacteria that are responsible for stopping the overgrowth of fungi in the intestine. Then be careful when you have overgrowths of fungi in your gut because many strange things will start happening to your body!

It's foolish never to take an antibiotic. Just, err on the conservative side. If there is a choice, do not take antibiotics. Instead, let your body's natural defenses try to take care of the problem first. If there is absolutely no choice, take the antibiotics as prescribed. Be sure to let your physician know that you do not want antibiotics unless absolutely medically necessary.

2 Weigh Yourself at Least Once a Day

Some people may tell you that you should not weigh yourself often. They'll tell you that it's a big distraction and it will not help you get to and keep your ideal weight.

I disagree. That philosophy is the same as telling people with high blood pressure that they shouldn't measure their blood pressure because it may distract them. It's essential to know what you weigh so you can determine your game plan.

I weigh myself several times each day. Over the years, I have learned about my body. I can predict what will happen if I don't get enough sleep, if I eat certain foods, or if I lay off exercise temporarily. It's important to have a good quality, accurate scale in your home and use it at least once a day. By using the scale, I have learned how to return to my ideal weight if I do gain a few pounds.

When I travel, I request a scale in my hotel room; hotels are often accommodating. Just ask.

3 Know Your BMI

You need to know your BMI, or Body Mass Index, to determine your ideal weight. Your BMI will indicate whether you are underweight, overweight, obese or at a healthy weight.

Here are the steps:
- **Multiply your weight in pounds by 703.**
- **Divide that answer by your height in inches.**
- **Divide that answer by your height in inches again.**

For example, a person who weighs 270 pounds and is 68 inches tall has a BMI of 41.0.

Here is the breakdown:

BMI	CATEGORY
Below 18.5	Underweight
18.5 - 24.9	Healthy
25.0 - 29.9	Overweight
30.0 - 39.9	Obese
Over 40.0	Morbidly Obese

If your BMI is 25.0 or greater, you need to make some changes. Think it's too late? It's not! It's never too late to make positive changes in your life.

④ Get Plenty of Sleep

Our lives are getting so busy we don't have enough hours in the day. To create more time, we decrease the number of hours we sleep.

Here's what happens to your body when you don't get enough sleep:

- Anxiety
- Chronic fatigue
- Compromised immune system
- Diabetes
- Heart disease
- High blood pressure
- Mood swings
- Weight gain

Most of us have different requirements for sleep. On the other hand, if you are averaging less than eight hours a night, there is a chance you are sleep deprived. Sleep is not a luxury. It is necessary to life and is as important as food and water.

5 Take a Yoga Class

Yoga keeps your body in tune. When you take a yoga class, you learn poses, stretches and breathing techniques that help you create and maintain a harmonious, finely tuned body. While a book is helpful, it's best to take a class because the instructor will guide you proper form and technique.

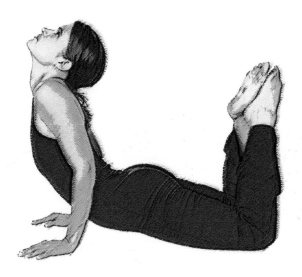

6 Vary Your Exercise!

Exercise along with diet can control stress, relax you, and help you eat better. Different exercises can improve bone density; reduce the risk of falls; lower the risk of heart disease, diabetes and high blood pressure; raise self-esteem; and reverse the natural muscle loss that occurs with aging.

I talked about walking in Day Two of this book. Once you get into the walking program and you are good about doing it every day, please feel free to mix in other types of aerobic exercise. Running and biking have always been two more of my favorites. Stair climbing, in-line skating and swimming are also fantastic. Give them all a try and see what you like.

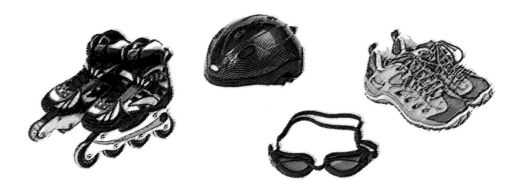

7 Meditate

Meditation can relieve stress and tension, as well as rejuvenate the mind, calm nerves and create a feeling of internal peace. If you don't know how to do it, read a book on meditation. There are tons of them.

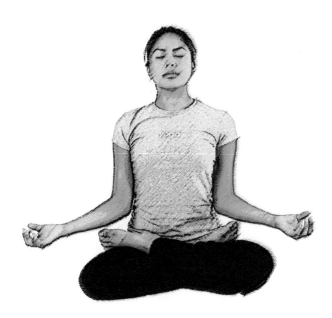

⑧ Get a Massage

Massage supports the healing process in the body, as well as improves blood circulation and helps remove toxins. The physical and emotional affects are life-affirming. A regularly scheduled weekly massage will make you feel like a new person.

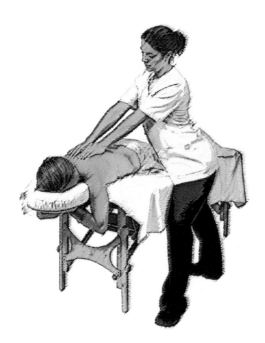

⑨ Floss Your Teeth

Seriously. Flossing results in healthier teeth and gums and prevents periodontal disease, which has been linked to cardiovascular disease. Also, while we are on the subject of teeth and gums, throw out your outdated toothbrush and begin using one of the electric brushes that remove plaque through sonic vibrations. These are sold everywhere and they are MUCH more effective than the standard toothbrush.

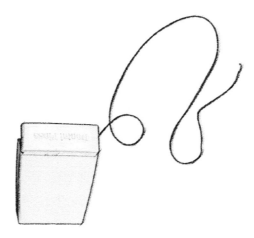

⬡10 Get Fitted for Orthotics

These custom soles correct and improve the way your feet hit the ground. They relieve alignment problems that can lead to foot, ankle, leg, hip and lower back pain. To assure that you get the proper evaluation and treatment, go to a podiatrist that is experienced in sports medicine.

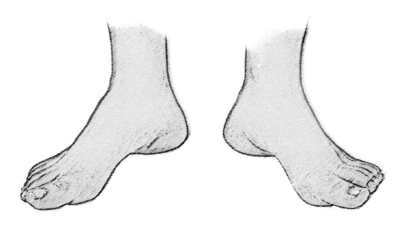

CONGRATULATIONS!

You have now finished reading the book that will change your life.

By reading this book, you've already made an investment in your best health. I urge you to get started right away. Unfortunately, it's easy to make excuses about why you cannot do this or why it won't work for you. It's far easier to keep doing the same thing you've always done.

If you follow this seven-day program, you will start noticing many positive, life-altering changes. The first day will put you in the right direction.

Return to Day One. Please reread the message. Once you reread it, promise yourself that you will say this message aloud every single day.

I have decided that
I will change my life.
In a short time
I will be thinner,
stronger, healthier,
younger looking
and more attractive.

I am ready to start!

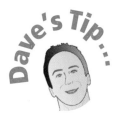

Dave's Tip...

Carry this book with you and refer back to it often. Keep the message in front of you. You can make it work.

Please understand that this will always be a "work in progress." I thought I was in good shape 10 years ago, but today I feel healthier and stronger than ever before. I am constantly discovering ways to improve. You can too. You are now on your way to becoming the healthiest, strongest and most beautiful person you have ever been.

Thank you for reading. I am committed to helping you reach your goal. Please visit davidmadow.com for more encouragement, ideas and coaching! Remember, you are no longer alone.

● For more information about the SEVEN DAYS please go to www.davidmadow.com.

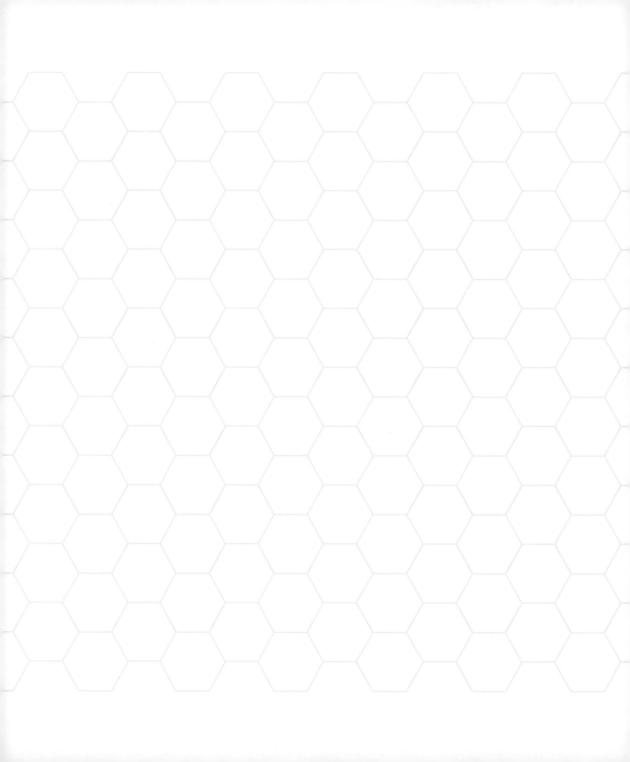

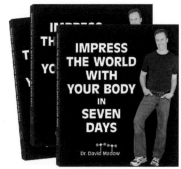

● To purchase additional copies of
**Impress the World With Your Body
in Seven Days**, please call **1-888-88-MADOW**
or go to **www.davidmadow.com**.

● Other titles available from Ridgemont Press
Is Your Frog Boiling? by Dr. Richard Madow

● For general information on our other products
or services, or to request information on how
you can have Dr. David Madow speak at your
next event, please contact The Madow Group at
1-888-88-MADOW or 1-410-526-4780 internationally.